WOMEN WITH ADHD

THE 7 SKILLS TO BE DEVELOPED WITH THIS LIFE-CHANGING GUIDE FOR THE QUEENS OF DISTRACTION WHO NOW CAN THRIVE IN A WORLD THAT WASN'T DESIGNED FOR THEM

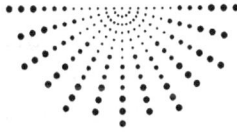

PATRICIA BLOOM

INTRODUCTION

ADHD is a neurobiological disease, which means it affects the biology of the central nervous and is characterized by impairments in executive functioning and self-control. Inattention, ADHD, or a mix of the two are the outcomes. To be diagnosed with ADHD, the condition must have begun in childhood and be causing impairment in one or more settings. Let's take a closer look at the consequences of executive dysfunction.

Every single one of us has struggled with the opening sentence of a dissertation or an essential letter at one point or another. The road to getting past the mental stalemate is not always smooth, but many of us eventually managed to summon this same complex planning and organizational skills required to write term papers or manage work projects or to plan a kitchen renovation or separate dark from the light-colored laundry at some point. The three kinds of

ADHD are ADD (often referred to as ADD or attention deficit disorder).

Though the overwhelming majority of instances of ADHD are hereditary, it is possible to develop ADHD as a result of brain damage, sickness, or perinatal exposure to harmful chemicals in rare circumstances. It's essential to remember ADHD isn't caused by bad parenting, too much TV, or a poor diet. We've probably heard the misconceptions about ADHD: "ADHD isn't real." "That child only needs a really good spanking," says the narrator. "Individuals having ADHD are simply lazy."

Despite breakthrough research and unambiguous neuro-biological results, many individuals continue to hold incorrect ideas about ADHD, and some even propagate outright falsehoods, which only serve to perpetuate confusion, shame and stigma. These misunderstandings and falsehoods regarding ADHD have existed since the disease itself; the detrimental impact on people's lives is quite real and extremely harmful. Find out the reality and equip yourself with evidence to counter the next ignorant remark about "poor parenting."

Behavioral problems (ADHD) affect two-thirds of children and will continue to affect them as adults. Although adults are calmer, they still struggle with organization and impulsivity. Some ADHD medicines for youngsters may help manage symptoms that persist into adulthood. ADHD's impact on sexuality may be difficult to quantify. This is because each person's sexual symptoms may vary. Sexual dysfunction may be caused by certain sexual symptoms. This may put a lot of strain on a relationship. Understanding how

ADHD impacts sexuality may help a couple of deal with stress in their relationship.

Women with ADHD have a hard time achieving orgasm. Some women claim to be able to have multiple orgasms in a short period, while others claim to be unable to achieve orgasm despite extended stimulation. Hypersensitivity is a possibility in people with ADHD. This implies that a sexual activity pleasurable to a partner who does not have ADHD may be annoying or uncomfortable to a person with ADHD.

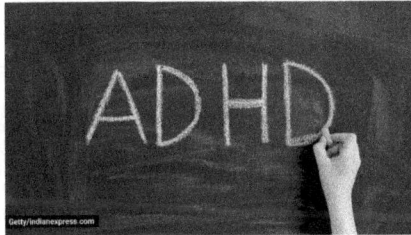

To someone with ADHD, how the smells feel and smell that often precede intercourse may be unpleasant or irritating. For someone with ADHD, hyperactivity is another barrier to intimacy. A companion with ADHD may find it difficult to relax sufficiently to be in the best of moods. The majority of instances with ADHD seem to be the consequence of aberrant brain development that begins before birth and leads to the atypical brain structure, inappropriate message transmission, and poor chemical activity inside the brain. Stimulant medications, the most successful therapy for ADHD, seem to have a normalizing impact, addressing the imbalance that is thought to cause ADHD symptoms, which is an essential insight into this aberrant biology. A parent of a newly diagnosed kid may blame oneself or their parenting, although the reason for the illness is more often than not unrelated to parenting. Parenting and the environment, on the other hand, may have a role in exacerbating the child's behavioral issues to some degree.

Approximately 80% of people with ADHD will be diagnosed with at least one additional mental illness at some point in their lives. Learning difficulties, anxiety, depression, sensory disorder, and conduct disorder are the most frequent ADHD comorbidities. Even though women and girls are now more often diagnosed with ADHD, women continue to encounter challenges getting an appropriate diagnosis. Only a few psychiatrists have been trained to diagnose women with ADHD. Because 95% of females having ADHD also have a coexisting illness including stress, anxiety, and bipolar disorder, their difficulties are frequently ascribed to their existing disease, whereas ADHD goes undiagnosed.

Another obstacle to female ADHD diagnosis is the absence of obvious symptoms of ADHD in childhood. To establish a diagnosis, current diagnostic standards need evidence of ADHD before the age of seven. Because females with ADHD are lesser prone to have been impulsive, disruptive, or rebellious as children, they are less prone to have been diagnosed with ADHD. Updated ADHD recommendations, set to be released in 2014, don't need early childhood symptoms. Many women will have to overcome this hurdle to identification until then.

Accepting your ADHD diagnosis, whether you've been diagnosed recently or for years, is a difficult job. You now have a reason why you do things the way you do, and even with the diagnoses, you still have many questions. How so many times have you heard someone remark, "If he wanted to, he could accomplish anything." There'd be no need for ADHD medicines, counseling, or other treatment options if this were the case. The world is a fantastic place to live. The truth is that it isn't that easy. It's essential to "want" to control your ADHD, but studies and experience show that even great desire isn't always enough.

It may be difficult to live with ADHD at times. Many people, on the other hand, are able to successfully control their ADHD symptoms and have productive, fulfilling lives. Based on the intensity of your problems, you may not require immediate medical attention. To gain a grip on your symptoms, you may make a variety of personal changes first.

Despite mounting irrefutable evidence, many individuals continue to deny whether ADHD is a legitimate medical disease. They use it as a justification to be sloppy or lazy. The fact that ADHD seems to come and go depending on the circumstances further adds to the skepticism of the skeptics. They say things like, "Why can't you get it together?" or "Why can't you pull it together?" Why can't you sit down and complete your schoolwork when you're OK with specific friends?"

Medications and counseling may help you manage the symptoms of ADHD. They aren't, however, your sole choices. Mindfulness meditation, in which you actively notice your moment-to-moment emotions and emotions, may now be a useful method to quiet your mind and increase your concentration, according to new research.

This technique is used by and over a third of people with ADHD, and approximately 40% of them rate it highly.

Mindfulness meditation, unlike other therapies, does not need medication or a visit to a doctor's office. It may be done while sitting, walking, or even doing certain kinds of yoga. Developing excellent everyday life management skills is an important part of gaining control of ADHD. These abilities will assist you in taking control of your everyday life, making effective usage of your time, learning how to break and achieve bigger life objectives, and developing daily routines that will improve well-being and decrease ADHD symptoms.

We should start developing these abilities while we are teenagers so that our shift to an independent life is easier. These abilities include knowing how to organize your time, prioritize and recall your daily chores, and also developing healthy daily routines such as getting enough sleep, exercising regularly, and eating properly. As an ADHD sufferer, your aim is to do all you can to enhance your brain's functioning, and sleep, diet, and exercise may help you achieve that goal by balancing your brain chemistry and improving your mood and concentration.

A healthy, well-balanced diet is essential for a happy & healthy existence. A balanced diet may help alleviate some of the symptoms of ADHD when used in conjunction with other treatments. Taking an objective look at your eating habits and determining what works well for you and your kid, on the other hand, maybe a difficult task. Eating correctly, as per the Centers for Disease and Prevention (CDC), may help reduce the risk of several chronic illnesses, especially heart disease. In addition, physical activity and exercise are advised as elements of a balanced lifestyle.

People often seek remedies for ADHD (attention deficit hyperactivity disorder) that people think will work in conjunction with and instead of the therapies prescribed by their doctor. Physicians and many others cure ADHD utilizing techniques that have been thoroughly researched, tested, and shown to be successful. Medication and behavioral therapy are two of these approaches. There are, however, a slew of alternative ADHD therapies that individuals hear about from colleagues or read about on the internet.

Adults with ADHD have a somewhat distinct appearance. It may manifest as agitation, disorganization, and difficulty concentrating. ADHD may also have some distinct advantages. Adult ADHD professionals may find that choosing a job that capitalizes on their abilities rather than relying primarily on weak spots is the key to a personal career. That, as well as effective ADHD therapy.

Listening carefully, being able to empathize with the person you're speaking to, and then acting in a helpful, non-defensive manner are all essential components of good communication. It also entails expressing your own ideas and emotions in a non-judgmental or accusatory manner so that your other partner can really hear and comprehend what you're saying rather than getting enraged or defensive. Stay calm, listen, empathize, react, and problem-solve; this may seem easy and uncomplicated. When emotions take control, however, excellent communication skills are frequently forgotten as partners participate in denials, accusations, refusals to resume talking, interruptions, and a variety of other behavior that obstruct healthy communication.

Adults with ADHD have even more communication difficulties since ADHD impulsivity may create disruptions even when emotions are low, and ADHD distractibility can cause your mind to wander just as your spouse is telling you something extremely important to him or her. As they're so focused on the ideas they are attempting to convey, somebody with ADHD may miss nonverbal signals that their companion is getting upset. Many people with ADHD have poor emotional self-control, making them highly and the over to even moderately unpleasant remarks. Those with ADHD may seem indifferent to their partner's demands while they are engrossed in the difficulties of their own everyday lives. It's awful to be late for work, a doctor's appointment, a meeting, a friend's birthday party, bringing the child to college, and much worse, picking them up from school. What can you do to break the cycle? How can you better manage your time? Experts say that successful planning requires two abilities that individuals with ADHD typically lack naturally but may learn: planning and timing.

1

BASICS OF ADHD

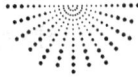

ADHD is a neurobiological disease, which means it affects the biology of the central nervous and is characterized by impairments in executive functioning and self-control. Inattention, ADHD, or a mix of the two are the outcomes. To be diagnosed with ADHD, the condition must have begun in childhood and be causing impairment in one or more settings. Let's take a closer look at the consequences of executive dysfunction.

Every single one of us has struggled with the opening sentence of a dissertation or an essential letter at one point or another. The road to getting past the mental stalemate is not always smooth, but many of us eventually managed to summon this same complex planning and organizational skills required to write term papers or manage work projects or to plan a kitchen renovation or separate dark from the light-colored laundry at some point. The three kinds of

ADHD are ADD (often referred to as ADD or attention deficit disorder).

Though the overwhelming majority of instances of ADHD are hereditary, it is possible to develop ADHD as a result of brain damage, sickness, or perinatal exposure to harmful chemicals in rare circumstances. It's essential to remember ADHD isn't caused by bad parenting, too much TV, or a poor diet. We've probably heard the misconceptions about ADHD: "ADHD isn't real." "That child only needs a really good spanking," says the narrator. "Individuals having ADHD are simply lazy."

These misunderstandings and falsehoods regarding ADHD have existed since the disease itself; the detrimental impact on people's lives is quite real and extremely harmful. Find out the reality and equip yourself with evidence to counter the next ignorant remark about "poor parenting." Despite breakthrough research and unambiguous neurobiological results, many individuals continue to hold incorrect ideas about ADHD, and some even propagate outright falsehoods, which only serve to perpetuate confusion, shame and stigma.

1.1 DEFINING ADHD

ADHD is a neurobiological disease, which means it affects the biology of the central nervous and is characterized by impairments in executive functioning and self-control. Inattention, ADHD, or a mix of the two are the outcomes. To be diagnosed with ADHD, the condition must have begun in childhood and be causing impairment in one or more settings. Let's take a closer look at the consequences of executive dysfunction.

Every single one of us has struggled with the opening sentence of a dissertation or an essential letter at one point or another. The road to getting past the mental stalemate is not always smooth, but many of us eventually managed to summon this same complex planning and organizational skills required to write term papers or manage work projects or to plan a kitchen renovation or separate dark from the light-colored laundry at some point. A collection of important mental activities that assist us in achieving our objectives is referred to as executive function (EF). These tasks include:

- Planning
- Strategizing
- Goal planning should be organized with careful consideration of key details.

Executive functioning, often known as the brain's control panel, is essentially concerned with finding out how to go from point A to point B to point C. It is analogous to the track that maintains the train on track when it stops, starts, or turns on its way to take you to your actual destination and on time.

Adults with attention deficit hyperactivity disorder (ADHD) typically:

- get distracted by stimuli and find it difficult to quit engaging and interesting actions and activities

- When beginning a project, don't pay attention to the instructions and often fail to keep pledges or obligations.
- Making choices based on impulse
- makes it difficult to enjoy peaceful leisure activities because they have difficulty completing things correctly when driving.

Because they affect almost every aspect of a woman's life, these symptoms represent the extent to which ADHD may be debilitating. While phrases such as "executive functioning" and "self-regulation" seem like they belong in a textbook, suffice to say that these apparently "absentminded" habits are brain-based, so there is a legitimate excuse for why you "do the things you do."

1.2 ADHD SUBTYPE TRIO

The three kinds of ADHD are ADD (often referred to as ADD or attention deficit disorder). Though the over-whelming majority of instances of ADHD are hereditary, it is possible to develop ADHD as a result of brain damage, sick-ness, or perinatal exposure to harmful chemicals in rare circumstances. It's essential to remember ADHD isn't caused by bad parenting, too much TV, or a poor diet. Following a review of the three kinds of ADHD, we'll go further into the symptoms.

- hyperactive/impulsive
- combined

- inattentive

The most frequent is the mixed subtype, which includes combined hyperactive/impulsive and inattentive symptoms, as the name implies. Let's take a look at each subtype and a few of the typical symptoms associated with it.

Hyperactive/Impulsive Subtype

The hyperactive/impulsive subtype of behavior is defined by excessive mental, verbal, or athletic activities that are often acted out without regard for the consequences. Most of the time, these habits are less noticeable in grownups than they are in children. In response to the following questions, consider if you show any of the behavior or tendencies described:

- Do you ever feel out of place in social situations?
- Do you find it difficult to complete a book?
- Do you have a habit of yelling things out and interrupting people, and you've been told you speak too much?
- During meetings, do you fidget by flicking your fingers or bouncing your feet?
- Do u find it very hard to unwind?
- Do you have a habit of overeating, overspending, and over-doing everything?
- Do you like high-intensity activities, even if they are potentially dangerous?
- Do you have a habit of leaving a trail or "stuff" behind you?

Although many people experience a few of these issues, individuals with ADHD experience them more often and tend to be more problematic in their daily lives. If you're experiencing many of these issues and they're interfering with your lifestyle, it may be necessary to be tested for ADHD.

Inattentive Subtype

In contrast to her hyperactive/impulsive counterpart, the woman with the attentive subtype of ADHD typically lives a calmer, more inward existence. She has a tendency to daydream, is always distracted, and worries or ruminates. Inattentive women may be physically lethargic or favor calm activities, but they can have hyperactive minds that need stimulus. It's critical to recognize that both kinds have similar symptoms.

We've all misplaced our keys or walked away from a dull discussion. If you experience many of the symptoms listed above and they're affecting your life, it's time to be tested for inattentive ADHD.

Combined Subtype

A woman with the mixed subtype of ADHD exhibits attention problems and irritability indicators, but not enough of either to be diagnosed with either subtype. She may be still on the go, but she also has a dreamy aspect to her personality, becoming lost in her thinking and overlooking little things in her job and life.

It's worth noting that few studies are trying to define the different subgroups of ADHD in men, and symptoms from all three categories may overlap. However, understanding what subtype you have may assist you and your medical team. Women with inattentive ADHD, for example, may be more likely to experience depression than their hyperactive/impulsive counterparts. Thus, practitioners should be particularly vigilant in searching for depression-related symptoms.

1.3 SYMPTOMS OF ADHD

Let's look at every one of them in more detail right now.

Impulsivity

What was the result? The new object appears on a table and remains there for weeks, decades, or longer until you get the opportunity to decide what to do next. By then, you've probably decided that you'd want to repair it. Now, you've lost the ticket. You discover someone at the shop and buy it, not understanding that you don't want it, don't have the room for that too, or, worse, possess two of that already. Lack of attention You find someone you like, similar to impulsive. Take, for instance, shoes, which you buy even though they don't go with anything in your wardrobe. Or you find a beautiful dresser at a yard sale for a great price; the ideal dresser for holding all the stuff you seem to accumulate but don't have a place for, but you forget that you have no room in your home to put the chest. Alternatively, you may be so engrossed in viewing the Morning Show each Thursday that you forget to take out the trash, which consisted of 3 weeks' worth of rubbish clogging up your garage.

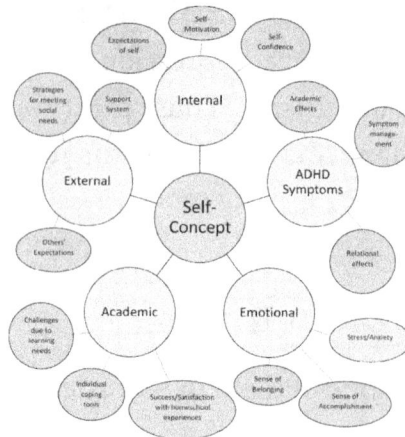

Difficulty Transitioning

An ADHD issue is the inability to shift from an enjoyable pastime to an unpleasant one, such as putting things away. This is just too dull to cope with for many women with Add. Decluttering the home is much less appealing than scrapbooking, playing a video game, or watching a movie. It's a double punch if your home is full of diversions. When you have a spouse and/or children, the clutter grows to tsunami dimensions as your attention is drawn in so many different ways.

Procrastination

Delay may also lead to clutter. It's there in front of you, eyeball to the eye, reminding you how tough it is to keep track of personal belongings. If you can't figure out what to store your things or set up the system for your stuff is too complicated or dull, and you just put it off, it will end up underfoot, perhaps permanently. Clutter occurs when you don't know what to do with items or while you have copies of items you previously had. Once you have an item on your hand and needs to be put away, you have a space where it belongs, thanks to creating a house for each of your belongings.

1.4 ADHD AND MYTHS

We've probably heard the misconceptions about ADHD: "ADHD isn't real." "That child only needs a really good spanking," says the narrator. "Individuals having ADHD are simply lazy." These misunderstandings and falsehoods regarding ADHD have existed since the disease itself; the detrimental impact on people's lives is quite real and extremely harmful. Find out the reality and equip yourself with evidence to counter the next ignorant remark about "poor parenting."

Despite breakthrough research and unambiguous neuro-biological results, many individuals continue to hold incorrect ideas about ADHD, and some even propagate outright falsehoods, which only serve to perpetuate confusion, shame and stigma. Here's where you can Understand the scientific facts about hyperactivity.

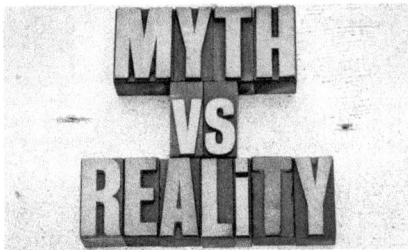

ADHD is not a recognized medical condition.

Major medical, psychiatric, as well as educational institutions have accepted ADHD as a valid diagnosis. In its Diagnostics and Diagnostic or statistical Manual, the real mental health "bible" using by doctors and psychologists, the American Psychological Association classifies ADHD as a medical condition. The biological basis of hyperactivity disorder may be found. It's thought to be caused by an overabundance of chemical signals in the brain, known as neurotransmitters. Inattention, impulsivity, and hyperactivity are the most common symptoms. ADHD, like other mental disorders, has no biological basis. This implies that scientists are still unsure about the biological foundation origins of ADHD, as well as the precise illness. The underlying pathology of diseases is widely established in most fields of medicine. Psychiatry, on the other hand, is an exception.

Drug corporations invented ADHD as a contemporary comedy.

ADHD isn't a new nor a uniquely American or Western problem. It's not conceived in reaction to pharmaceutical business demands or contemporary academic constraints, and the need to excel in school.

Now, they are serious issues and factors that may lead to an overdiagnosis of ADHD. However, these events do not completely explain ADHD. You may find accounts of youngsters that appear quite similar to Kids with ADHD in medical literature dating back a century. That exact diagnosis didn't exist a generation back, but doctors described youngsters who were impulsive, hyperactive and inattentive, all of the characteristics that we now associate with ADHD. Few of the first accounts date as far back as the 1700s.

We have knowledge through observational studies of ADHD occurrence, in which researchers survey a lot of babies in various areas across the globe to determine the prevalence of ADHD. This has been accomplished in the African countries, as well as in South America, Asia, Europe and North America. And it demonstrates ADHD is a global problem.

Furthermore, the prevalence of ADHD is also pretty constant throughout the globe, ranging from around 5% to 6% of the population. Where ADHD is only a Western issue, we would observe extremely high rates in Europe And North America and comparatively lower rates in the rest of the world. It is not what evidence indicates.

Diagnosis Process

In addition, there are no objective diagnostic tests for ADHD that can establish whether or not a person has the condition. Symptom assessments and other metrics are being used by physicians to identify ADHD symptomology.

In the meanwhile, as scientists strive to develop biological validity and accurate screening procedures, there are other methods to be comfortable in an ADHD diagnosis. The first is via a concept known as dependability among scientists. This relates to the capacity of two physicians to assess the same kid and arrive at the same conclusion independently.

The diagnosis of ADHD is highly accurate. It is, in reality, one of the most accurate diagnoses in the field of psychiatry, particularly in the field of child psychiatry. The accuracy of identifying ADHD with a chest radiograph is comparable to that of identifying tuberculosis with a chest X-ray. This is really remarkable.

Bad Parenting causes ADHD.

The issue is caused by a change in brain chemicals rather than a lack of discipline. It's not because a kid with ADHD says anything or jumps out of the seat in school because he is still not trained that these actions are inappropriate. He can't control his urges, that's why.

Extremely strict upbringing, which may include punishing a kid for actions he has no control of, may aggravate ADHD. Typically, expert treatments such as medication therapy, counseling, and behavior modification therapy and others are needed.

Only boys are affected by ADHD.

Girls are equally as likely as boys to develop ADHD, and the symptoms produced by the condition are unaffected by gender. Boys, however, are more prone than females to be identified as a result of this misconception.

ADHD is a disorder that children outgrow with time

And over 70% of those who are identified with ADHD as a kid also have it as an adolescent. Up to half of those who have it as a child will stay to have ADHD as adults. Although it is believed that 5-6% of both the elderly have ADHD, the great majority of people go untreated, with just one out of every four seeking treatment.

Adults diagnosed with ADHD, on the other hand, are very susceptible to mood problems, anxiety, and drug addiction if they do not get treatment. They often face challenges in their careers, financial and legal issues, and strained personal relationships.

A kid who can play video games for hours couldn't possibly have ADHD

It's not uncommon for a kid with ADHD to be easily distracted in one situation but laser-focused in another.

What is the reason behind this? Since ADHD does not imply a lack of focus. ADHD is a word that applies to a lack of control over one's attention. Hyperfocus may be induced by extremely facilitate timely or activities. It's in the more ordinary and less exciting situations that distractibility truly shines through.

When kids use ADHD medication, they are much more prone to abuse drugs as adolescents.

In fact, it's the polar opposite. Untreated ADHD raises the likelihood of a person abusing alcohol or drugs. This risk may be reduced with the right therapy. It is undeniably true that youngsters with ADHD are actually more prone to misuse drugs than neurotypical kids. This impact, however, is not caused by the usage of the medicine. Long-term studies comparing students with ADHD who take medication versus ADHD children who do not take medication have shown this. Researchers observe them throughout time and discover that those who take medication have no higher risk of drug addiction than those who do not take medication for ADHD.

Furthermore, throughout the course of far more than 50 years of usage, the medicines used to manage ADHD are shown to be effective and safe. These medications do not cure ADHD, although they are quite successful in alleviating its symptoms. This misunderstanding stems from a fairly frequent blunder: confusing correlation with the disease causation. The fact is that ADHD, not really the medicine, is what raises the risk of drug abuse.

Kids who are provided with extra concessions due to their ADHD have an undue advantage.

In fact, kids struggling with ADHD are in a disadvantageous position, and modifications, school policies, and disability education laws attempt to mitigate this disadvantage to the greatest extent feasible. ADHD is actually quite a valid and important condition. Studies show clearly that having ADHD puts you at the chance for a variety of bad outcomes, as not finishing high school, leaving college, adolescent pregnancies, automobile accidents, and other issues.

The government Special education Law (IDEA) attempts to mitigate these dangers by mandating public schools to meet the unique needs and requirements of all disabled children, including those who have ADHD. Special adjustments, such as additional time on exams, merely level the field, allowing kids with ADHD to learn just as well as their peers.

ADHD People are lazy

Many famous, high-achieving people in the past, such as Mozart, Franklin Roosevelt, Abe Lincoln, Salvador Dali and George Herbert Mead, are believed to have had ADHD. Richard Branson, CEO Virgin, is among the high-achieving individuals with ADHD in business today.

Many females with untreated ADHD grow up and hearing themselves branded as "spacey," "far too chatty," and "disorganized," which is a worrisome fact. Even if their unhappy parents and instructors know these young ladies are bright and competent, they may lag behind academically as teens. Even as adults, many people face challenges as a result of increasing responsibilities and new jobs.

In an era when people are increasingly conscious of income inequalities and societal injustices, academics are focusing more on health disparities like this one: Boys continue to be identified with ADHD at a significantly higher rate than girls. Is it just the case that males suffer from ADHD more frequently than girls? Researchers are increasingly discovering that it is more complicated than that.

1.5 HOW SEX AFFECTS ADHD SUBTYPES AND DIAGNOSIS

ADHD is referred to as a psychiatric condition that impairs one's ability or capability to do any of the following tasks:

- remain organized
- manage schedules
- remember things
- sit still
- control urges
- pay close attention, concentrate for extended amounts of time
- notice certain details
- divide tasks and objectives into sections or stages

Symptoms associated with ADHD usually fall under three subtypes:

Inattentive

It is defined as the inability to concentrate, being quickly distracted, often misplacing important things and making many thoughtless errors,

Hyperactive/Impulsive

Restlessness, trouble staying sat, excessive chatting, and frequent interruptions are all signs of hyperactivity/impulsivity.

Combined

Both attentive and hyperactivity symptoms describe combined. Females may be underdiagnosed, according to some studies, since they exhibit more signs of inattentive ADHD than hyperactive/impulsive ADHD. The relatively quiet distractibility of attentive ADHD does not attract the attention of families, teachers, and health professionals as easily as the characteristics of hyperactive/impulsive ADHD, which may be louder and more disruptive. A person must exhibit at least five to six of the nine main symptoms specified in DSM-5 for a particular form of ADHD to obtain an ADHD diagnosis. These symptoms are occurring and being disruptive to daily life over the past six months and in more places than one, for example, at home or at school.

1.6 HOW SEX INFLUENCES ADHD SYMPTOMS

The signs and symptoms of ADHD differ between individuals. Sweeping generalizations gender-based aren't always useful in ensuring that each person receives the best possible treatment. Here's what a new study on gender disparities in symptoms of ADHD has been discovered.

Hormones and ADHD

Changes in hormonal changes may affect ADHD symptoms in both men and women. When sex hormones affect physical symptoms and behavior, people of both genders may notice a change in symptoms nearing puberty. Hormone fluctuations may influence symptoms in a variety of ways, including:

- Hormone fluctuations during menopause and pregnancy may exacerbate symptoms.
- After your menstrual cycle's ovulation period, your inattention may grow.
- Fluctuations in estrogen levels during your period may exacerbate symptoms of ADHD, especially in females having ADHD who are prone to impulsivity.

1.7 HOW SEX AND GENDER CAN AFFECT TREATMENT

Doctors often give stimulant or non-stimulant medicines to children and adolescents who have been diagnosed with ADHD in order to control symptoms and enhance functioning. According to studies, physicians give fewer medicines to girls having ADHD in comparison with men with ADHD. This disparity in prescribing rates is puzzling since research indicates that both amphetamine and non-stimulant medicines help females as much or even more than boys with most symptoms. Again, these disparities may be explained by differences in behavior between boys and girls, which could lead to males receiving more therapy than girls.

Medication rates are rather evenly distributed among adults. Women are still prescribed less medicine than males, although the disparity is less pronounced. More study is needed to understand how men's and women's bodies absorb ADHD medicines, as well as how increasing and decreasing hormones affect medication efficacy. Stimulant drugs, for example, have been found in tests to "wear off" sooner during the day in females. Understanding these variations may aid physicians in tailoring therapy to the specific requirements of each woman. Medications aren't the sole option for treating ADHD. Cognitive-behavioral therapy, Psychotherapy, and social skill training may also be beneficial.

Women and girls should speak with therapists and counselors about any additional dangers they may face, according to health professionals. According to research, women and girls with ADHD are at larger risk of developing drug abuse issues, risky behavior, self-harming and unhealthy eating. Women and girls who are educated about ADHD are more prepared to avoid:

- self-blaming and feelings of guilt
- seeking potentially harmful stimulation
- coping methods that can cause more damage than improvement

Why does an early diagnosis matter?

People can have had worse results throughout their lives if a clear prognosis and treatments available are delayed, including:

- less professional and vocational achievement
- more conflicted partnerships
- expensive healthcare
- more anxiety/stress
- low self-esteem
- health symptoms like abdominal distress and migraine
- sleeping problems

Whenever it is about ADHD, females are often misdiagnosed or underdiagnosed. It's possible they've become better at adjusting for or concealing their symptoms. It may also be that mothers, health care providers and teachers are less likely to notice signs of inattention than they are for louder and upsetting symptoms. Women are also more prone to:

- have variable symptoms due to hormones
- develop effective anxiety symptoms and depression
- have poorer self-esteem
- greater interpersonal conflict

For the time being, here's something to think about. You are not a slacker if you have ADHD. You aren't a scatterbrain.

You have a psychological problem that makes it 4.5 percent of people in the US difficult to pay much attention, controlling urges, planning, organizing, and finishing activities difficult or impossible. It's like turning tapestries upon the art side to get the proper sort of treatment. The tangles and threads may start to make sense, and it can be very lovely.

1.8 ADHD IN ADULTHOOD: THE SIGNS YOU NEED TO KNOW

According to the Psychiatric Association, (ADHD) affects 8.7% of kids and 2.6 percent of us adults (APA). According to the Medical Research Council, the figures may be much higher. Many girls and women who have the disease are also undiagnosed. Untreated ADHD may manifest itself as environmental and biological issues that disrupt a person's everyday life, especially their relationships. Adult ADHD symptoms must be recognized in order to get appropriate therapy. Continue reading to discover more about these signs and symptoms.

Lack of focus

The most telling sign of ADHD includes a lack of concentration that goes beyond just being unable to pay attention. It also implies:

- being quickly distracted
- having difficulty listening to people in a discussion
- missing details
- failing to complete assignments or initiatives

Hyperfocus is the polar opposite of lack of focus.

Hyperfocus

People with ADHD, according to a tiny 2020 research, are easily distracted. They may also suffer from a condition known as hyperfocus. An individual with ADHD may get so absorbed in something which they lose track of everything else going on around them. It's much easy to lose sight of time and disregard people around you when you're focused like this. This may lead to misconceptions in relationships.

Disorganization

Everyone's life may be difficult at times. However, compared to someone that doesn't have ADHD, somebody with ADHD has more difficult life situations. This may make it tough for them all to keep track of everything. It may be difficult for adults with ADHD to control their organizing abilities. This may involve difficulties keeping track of activities and properly prioritizing them.

2

SCIENCE OF ADHD AND MORE

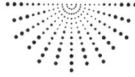

Behavioral problems (ADHD) affect two-thirds of children and will continue to affect them as adults. Although adults are calmer, they still struggle with organization and impulsivity. Some ADHD medicines for youngsters may help manage symptoms that persist into adulthood. ADHD's impact on sexuality may be difficult to quantify. This is because each person's sexual symptoms may vary. Sexual dysfunction may be caused by certain sexual symptoms. This may put a lot of strain on a relationship. Understanding how ADHD impacts sexuality may help a couple of deal with stress in their relationship.

Women with ADHD have a hard time achieving orgasm. Some women claim to be able to have multiple orgasms in a short period, while others claim to be unable to achieve orgasm despite extended stimulation.

Hypersensitivity is a possibility in people with ADHD.

This implies that a sexual activity pleasurable to a partner who does not have ADHD may be annoying or uncomfortable to a person with ADHD. To someone with ADHD, the smells feel and smell that often precede intercourse may be unpleasant or irritating. For someone with ADHD, hyperactivity is another barrier to intimacy. A companion with ADHD may find it difficult to relax sufficiently to be in the best of moods. The majority of instances with ADHD seem to be the consequence of aberrant brain development that begins before birth and leads to the atypical brain structure, inappropriate message transmission, and poor chemical activity inside the brain.

Stimulant medications, the most successful therapy for ADHD, seem to have a normalizing impact, addressing the imbalance that is thought to cause ADHD symptoms, which is an essential insight into this aberrant biology. A parent of a newly diagnosed kid may blame oneself or their parenting, although the reason for the illness is more often than not unrelated to parenting. Parenting and the environment, on the other hand, may have a role in exacerbating the child's behavioral issues to some degree.

Approximately 80% of people with ADHD will be diagnosed with at least one additional mental illness at some point in their lives. Learning difficulties, anxiety, depression, sensory disorder, and conduct disorder are the most frequent ADHD comorbidities. Is it possible to grow out of ADD? Cured? ADHD was formerly thought to be a childhood disease that diminished with maturity. That is not the case. Two-thirds of children with ADHD grow up to be adults with the disorder. Many people who were identified with ADHD as children believe that adulthood has helped them overcome their symptoms.

What does the study say about this? Researchers are still looking into the possibility that some individuals surpass ADHD and at least the majority of its outward signs. Nevertheless, about 80% of young individuals with ADHD will remain to have it throughout adulthood. This implies that roughly 20% of people who were labeled with ADHD as kids will no more fit the medical criteria.

2.1 ADHD: CHILDHOOD TO ADULTHOOD

Behavioral problems (ADHD) affect two-thirds of children and will continue to affect them as adults. Although adults are calmer, they still struggle with organization and impulsivity. Some ADHD medicines for youngsters may help manage symptoms that persist into adulthood.

Effects of ADHD on Sexuality

ADHD's impact on sexuality may be difficult to quantify. This is because each person's sexual symptoms may vary. Sexual dysfunction may be caused by certain sexual symptoms. This may put a lot of strain on a relationship. Understanding how ADHD impacts sexuality may help a couple of deal with stress in their relationship. Sadness, emotional immaturity, and anxiety are all typical symptoms of ADHD. All of these factors may have an adverse effect on sexual desire. Maintaining order and structure, for example, maybe tiring for someone with ADHD. They may lack the motivation or energy to participate in sexual activities.

Hypersexuality and hyposexuality are two sexual symptoms associated with ADHD. If an individual with ADHD has sexual problems, they may fit into such two groups. It's also worth noting that sexual symptoms aren't included in the American Psychiatric Association's accepted diagnostic criteria for ADHD.

Hyposexuality and ADHD

An individual's sex drive plummets, and they frequently lose interest in sexual activities, which is the polar opposite of hypersexuality. This may be a result of the ADHD itself. It may also occur as a secondary effect of medicine, especially antidepressants, often given to individuals with ADHD and other attention deficit hyperactivity disorders.

For someone with ADHD, sexual activity is no different than any other activity that presents difficulty. They may have difficulty focusing during sex, lose all interest in what they're doing, or get distracted from their sexual activity.

Hypersexuality and ADHD

You have an abnormally strong sex desire if you are hypersexual. Sexual arousal produces endorphins and activates neurotransmitters in the brain. This creates a sense of serenity, which helps to alleviate the restlessness that is frequently associated with ADHD. Promiscuity and pornographic usage, on the other hand, may cause relationship problems. It's essential to remember that promiscuity or the usage of pornography isn't part of the ADHD diagnosis criteria.

Due to impulsive issues, some individuals with ADHD can engage in hazardous sexual behavior. People with ADHD are also more likely to develop drug abuse problems, impair decision-making and lead to sexual risk-taking.

2.2 OVERCOMING SEXUAL CHALLENGES

Women with ADHD have a hard time achieving orgasm. Some women claim to be able to have multiple orgasms in a short period, while others claim to be unable to achieve orgasm despite extended stimulation.

Hypersensitivity is a possibility in people with ADHD. This implies that a sexual activity pleasurable to a partner who does not have ADHD may be annoying or uncomfortable to a person with ADHD.

To someone with ADHD, the smells feel and smell that often precede intercourse may be unpleasant or irritating. For someone with ADHD, hyperactivity is another barrier to intimacy. A companion with ADHD may find it difficult to relax sufficiently to be in the best of moods.

Mix it up

Bored in the bedroom may be reduced by experimenting with different positions, places, and methods. Before sex, talk about ways to spice it up so that both parties feel at ease.

Prioritize

Practice being present in the moment. Remove all distractions and attempt soothing yoga poses or meditation with your partner. Make sex dates and stick to them. You won't get distracted if you make sex a priority.

Communicate and compromise

Discuss how having ADHD may impact your sexual expression and intimacy. Be mindful of your partner's requirements if they have ADHD. If they're light-sensitive or strong scents, for instance, turn off lights and avoid using lotions or fragrances.

Don't be scared to seek professional assistance from a sex therapist. Couples counseling and sex therapy are very beneficial to many couples dealing with ADHD.

2.3 THE CAUSATIVE FACTORS OF ADHD

The majority of instances with ADHD seem to be the consequence of aberrant brain development that begins before birth and leads to the atypical brain structure, inappropriate message transmission, and poor chemical activity inside the brain. Stimulant medications, the most successful therapy for ADHD, seem to have a normalizing impact, addressing the imbalance that is thought to cause ADHD symptoms, which is an essential insight into this aberrant biology.

The degree of a child's issues may be influenced by how he is handled and nurtured, but it cannot cause the problem. Certain methods of childrearing may exacerbate the issue, while others may alleviate it. No kind of parenting, even borderline abusive parenting, can cause ADHD in a kid who is not predisposed to it. Because childrearing methods may influence the severity of an ADHD child's issues to some extent, changes in these methods are generally beneficial. Even while such psychological methods may aid in treating ADHD children, the root of their problems is physiological and inborn. Some people believe that an ADHD child's conduct is caused by a lack of control, a chaotic home life, or too much television since attention deficit disorder (ADHD) symptoms impair a children's ability to study or get along with others.

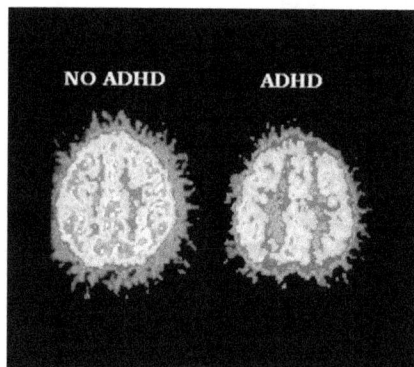

A parent of a newly diagnosed kid may blame oneself or their parenting, although the reason for the illness is more often than not unrelated to parenting. Parenting and the environment, on the other hand, may have a role in exacerbating the child's behavioral issues to some degree.

2.4 GENETICS OF ADHD

It's hardly surprising that ADHD runs in families. Since we all know, children have temperamental variances from birth. Children vary from each other from the time they are born until they reach preadolescence, according to studies, because some of those differences are linked to behavioral issues as the kid gets older. The challenges that an ADHD kid is likely to have at birth (colic, feeding issues, and sleeping issues, for example) are most likely the consequence of inborn temperamental abnormalities.

Furthermore, it is a well-known fact that certain temperaments prefer to run in the family. Some families have high-strung children, while others have calmer youngsters. There is no such thing as an all-or-nothing temperamental trait. It's akin to being tall. From the extremely small to the very tall, there are various kinds of heights.

Although being 4' 6" or 7' 2" tall may be uncomfortable, most extremely small or very high individuals do not have a sickness. Similarly, most levels of high-strangeness aren't harmful until they're extreme. All of the characteristics we've examined in relation to ADHD youngsters are present in all children. All children, at times, have attention spans, are bored, and are irritable when they don't receive what they want. These traits are present in ADHD youngsters to a significant degree. They are, in a way, the opposites of the ordinary, like extremely short or really tall individuals. They have an excess of and a deficiency of some typical features.

When we talk to parents whose children have ADHD, they often tell us that they experienced similar issues when their son or daughter was age. Depending on the circumstances, being aware of this resemblance may be beneficial or detrimental. When parents recall the issues they encountered and the methods that were most effective in dealing with them, it may be beneficial.

This may offer valuable information for assisting the kid. When parents downplay the problems caused by ADHD, the knowledge may be detrimental. If the parent is reluctant to admit (even to themselves) that ADHD has caused (or continues to cause) them difficulties, the child's problems may be minimized. If this occurs, the parents may overlook significant issues with their kids that need attention.

2.5 RISK FACTORS OF ADHD

There have been no definitive reasons for a child's ADHD to be discovered. However, the following variables may increase the chance of developing the disease:-

Altered anatomy or function of the brain

Brain scans have revealed that adults and children with ADHD have distinct brain regions, particularly those linked to movement and attention spans. According to several research, individuals with ADHD have a different frontal lobe (located at the front of the brain). This topic is about making decisions. Neurons like dopamine and dopamine may also be out of whack in the brain. These neurotransmitters are the brain's chemical messengers.

Maternal drug abuse, alcohol intake and smoking

According to some research, pregnant cigarette smokers who drink alcohol or use illicit drugs are more likely to give birth to a child who later has attention deficit hyperactivity disorder (ADHD). The precise pathophysiology that is responsible for this relationship is not fully understood. However, it is hypothesized that this kind of maltreatment in utero or inside the womb decreases neuronal activity and changes the neurotransmitters, which are nerve messenger chemicals. Expectant mothers linked to environmental pollutants are at risk of having a baby to children who may develop attention deficit hyperactivity disorder (ADHD).

3

WOMEN WITH ADHD

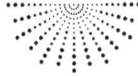

Even though women and girls are now more often diagnosed with ADHD, women continue to encounter challenges getting an appropriate diagnosis. Only a few psychiatrists have been trained to diagnose women with ADHD. Because 95% of females having ADHD also have a coexisting illness including stress, anxiety, and bipolar disorder, their difficulties are frequently ascribed to their existing disease, whereas ADHD goes undiagnosed. Another obstacle to female ADHD diagnosis is the absence of obvious symptoms of ADHD in childhood. To establish a diagnosis, current diagnostic standards need evidence of ADHD before the age of seven. Because females with ADHD are lesser prone to have been impulsive, disruptive, or rebellious as children, they are less prone to have been diagnosed with ADHD. Updated ADHD recommendations, set to be released in 2014, don't need early childhood symptoms.

Many women will have to overcome this hurdle to identification until then.

Do you imagine a hyperactive young kid climbing the walls when you think of someone with ADHD? Quite a few individuals do. However, this isn't the full picture. ADHD may also manifest itself in the form of a 30-year-old lady securely planted on the sofa. Women with ADHD have a particular list of symptoms and difficulties and coping with the typical pleasures of the disease. Understanding them may help you feel less guilty and confused about being an untidy little woman in a society that demands perfection. When women learn they have dyslexia, they often feel relieved (ADHD). They may have hated themselves for their failures for years, and their consciousness has suffered as a result. Emotional, mental, and bodily fatigue may have resulted from their constant concern over every aspect of their life.

They have an answer now that they have been diagnosed with ADHD, and they recognize that their illnesses are not their fault. Feelings of inadequacy may go away once individuals understand they have ADHD, putting them in a good situation to effectively manage their symptoms.

3.1 WOMEN AND ADHD

For decades, the bulk of ADHD literature and research centered on boys, and boys were the bulk of children sent to centers for ADHD assessments. In the mid-1990s, there was a gradual increase in interest in women and girls with ADHD.

Adult ADHD clinics, which first opened their doors in

the mid-1990s, reported a significantly greater woman to man ratio than kid ADHD clinics had previously recorded. Girls had to rely on instructors and parents to send them for assessment and treatment, while women may seek therapy independently. Most of these females, identified as having ADHD for the initial time in their 30s and later, said they had been seeking therapy for years but had been misdiagnosed with anxiety instead of ADHD.

Even though women and girls are now more often diagnosed with ADHD, women continue to encounter challenges getting an appropriate diagnosis. Only a few psychiatrists have been trained to diagnose women with ADHD. Because 95% of females having ADHD also have a coexisting illness including stress, anxiety, and bipolar disorder,

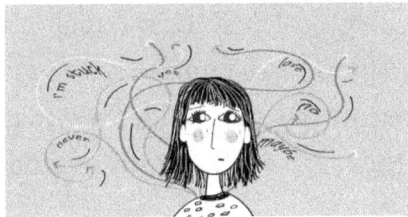

their difficulties are frequently ascribed to their existing disease, whereas ADHD goes undiagnosed. Another obstacle to female ADHD diagnosis is the absence of obvious symptoms of ADHD in childhood. To establish a diagnosis, current diagnostic standards need evidence of ADHD before the age of seven. Because females with ADHD are lesser prone to have been impulsive, disruptive, or rebellious as children, they are less prone to have been diagnosed with ADHD. Updated ADHD recommendations, set to be released in 2014, don't need early childhood symptoms. Many women will have to overcome this hurdle to identification until then.

3.2 WHY GIRLS AND WOMEN ARE UNDER-DIAGNOSED

Boys are more likely than females to be diagnosed with ADHD for a variety of reasons. Here are a few of the most important factors:

- ADHD manifests itself in various ways in different individuals. The main symptoms may be influenced by sex, gender, and hormones.
- Gender stereotypes may prevent instructors from identifying signs of ADHD in female students. Because symptoms in females may be milder, doctors may be hesitant to identify them with ADHD if they also exhibit signs of emotional problems.
- Because most research has focused on males until recently, more is understood about how guys suffer from ADHD and how it affects their life.
- Gender norms may drive females to conceal and disguise ADHD symptoms. Stereotypes about neatness, organization, collaboration, compliance, and social behavior may lead girls and women in schools and family systems to ignore or adjust for ADHD symptoms.

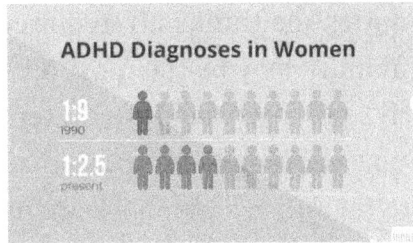

ADHD Diagnoses in Women

1:9 1990

1:2.5 present

3.3 STRUGGLES OF WOMEN WITH ADHD

Do you imagine a hyperactive young kid climbing the walls when you think of someone with ADHD? Quite a few individuals do. However, this isn't the full picture. ADHD may also manifest itself in the form of a 30-year-old lady securely planted on the sofa. Women with ADHD have a particular list of symptoms and difficulties and coping with the typical pleasures of the disease. Understanding them may help you feel less guilty and confused about being an untidy little woman in a society that demands perfection. These are just a few of the hidden difficulties of a lady with ADHD, in case you didn't know.

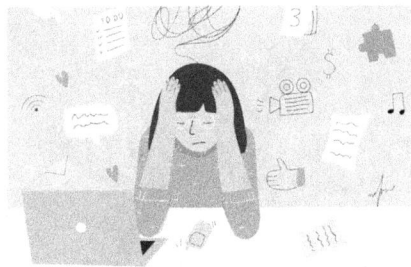

Internalizing others' judgments leads to self-blame
A battle with her tremendous feeling of inadequacy in

performing the duties she thinks are required of her by her parents and community may be the most difficult issue for a female with ADHD. Girls are taught to "internalize" negative criticism, apologize, comply, not push back, and accept responsibility. On the other hand, boys are usually taught to "externalize" – to fight when they are assaulted, to view the issue as something external to them.

Hormonal fluctuations

Hormonal changes that begin at adolescence continue to have a significant impact on the lives of females with ADHD. Their monthly hormonal changes aggravate the difficulties they face as a result of their ADHD. Several women say that the anxiety of being the main parent of kids having ADHD while also struggling with their ADHD approaches emergency levels every month during their menstrual period, which may last up to a week. Although the proportion of older women with ADHD has yet to be determined, it is fair to anticipate that hormonal changes linked with menopause will increase ADHD signs of emotional reactivity once again.

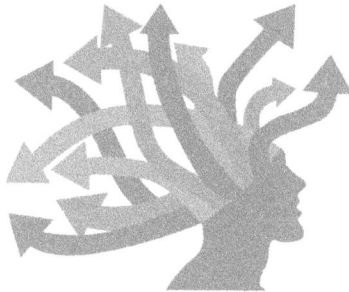

Low estrogen levels have been linked to decreased cognitive performance, particularly poor auditory recall and word retrieval, in addition to PMS. These intellectual deficits, along with the impaired executive performance observed in ADHD, can serve as a trigger for referring older females who were formerly able to operate at a high level earlier to the low estrogen condition linked with early menopause.

Instead of having a support system, Become a support system

Women are often cast in the position of caregivers, both at work and home. While males with ADHD are usually encouraged to surround themselves with a support system, few women have such access, and society has historically expected women to provide the support system.

The rise of "dual-career couples" has exacerbated the difficulties faced by women with ADHD. During most of the last two decades, an increasing number of women have been expected to perform the more conventional duties of mother and wife and work effectively and relentlessly while juggling the responsibilities of a full-time job.

Single parenting

In the United States, the rate of divorce is close to 50% of all marriages. If ADHD is introduced to the number of marital stresses, divorce becomes much more probable. Following a divorce, women are overwhelmingly left as main caregivers for their children. When you combine ADHD with the enormous responsibility of single parenthood, the consequence is chronic fatigue, emotional depletion, and sometimes tremendous disarray, as a female with ADHD is forced to balance a set of duties that would be difficult for any person much alone one with ADHD.

Boobs, periods, and ADHD

Girls with ADHD have an uphill fight from the start. Because the symptoms of ADHD in girls vary from those in males, they are more likely to go undiagnosed or misdiagnosed.

Because evidently boobs, menstrual periods, and eyeliner aren't enough to hurl at a middle schooler, symptoms in females generally emerge around the beginning of puberty.

Unless you're like me and have both, ADHD often manifests itself in women as symptoms of inattention rather than hyperactivity. As a result, our inattention is often dismissed as a character defect rather than a curable illness.

School Daze

When females with ADHD enter college and are no longer surrounded by the rigidity of their parents, curfews, and obligatory school attendance, things start to become interesting. Women with ADHD, for example, are known to be the quick life of the party while having a nervous breakdown on the inside over the ever-growing mound of schoolwork they haven't even begun to do.

Taking care of their children while neglecting oneself

A female with ADHD should concentrate on therapy for herself when she wants to be the perfect mom for her kid, much as normal flight instructions urge parents to put on their personal oxygen masks before helping their child. Helping children with ADHD operate better involves their parents' full involvement in understanding and regularly using excellent parenting methods, establishing home schedules, and educating the kid to see his ADHD as a positive, productive problem-solving tool. Consequently, the best approach for a mother having ADHD to assist her kid is to get herself treated and educated about ADHD.

Manic pixie nightmare

According to research, women who have ADHD have an unpleasant propensity to keep their issues (and their dishes) to themselves, keeping no one in the loop about the turmoil and worry that is steadily taking over their lives. This may be because they never got a proper diagnosis and thus did not have recourse to the medicines and coping techniques that would be beneficial. Even though you are completely aware of the fact that you will have ADHD, it is very easy to get consumed by feelings of guilt when you have fallen behind with your obligations.

And, regrettably, the society in which we live still places more expectations on women in some areas. Guess you forgot to send your friend a birthday card this year? Is it possible that you were distracted when your buddy wanted you to pay close attention? And you're a lady who has failed.

Girl probs in a man's world

According to research, women who have ADHD have an unpleasant propensity to keep their issues (and their dishes) to themselves, keeping no one in the loop about the turmoil and worry that is steadily taking over their lives. It's possible that this is due to the fact that they never got a proper diagnosis and thus did not have recourse to the medicines and coping techniques that would be beneficial. Even though you are completely aware that you will have ADHD, it is very easy to get consumed by feelings of guilt when you have fallen behind with your obligations.

And, regrettably, the society in which we live still places more expectations on women in some areas. Guess you forgot to send your friend a birthday card this year? Is it possible that you were distracted when your buddy wanted you to pay close attention? And you're a lady who has failed.

Having it all' with ADHD

If you're a female with ADHD, the greatest thing you can do for yourself (apart from medicine and organizing techniques) is to take a break. Thank your brain for all it can accomplish and set reasonable objectives for everything else. Also, don't be embarrassed to brag about your ADHD. We may be grown women with homes, vehicles, and banking information, but we have the same right to be distracted as the children.

3.4 PSYCHOLOGICAL AND EMOTIONAL EFFECTS OF ADHD ON WOMEN

- Several studies have shown that females with ADHD have poorer self-esteem than boys with ADHD, even into adulthood.
- A study comparing girls with ADHD to girls without ADHD found that females with ADHD

had more difficulty in their social interactions than girls without ADHD.

- Research on women and girls indicates that women with ADHD are more likely to have symptoms similar to those of illnesses, including melancholy, stress, and disordered eating. Additionally, women who have been previously or simultaneously identified with ADHD, hyperactive/impulsive type, are more likely to have a borderline personality disorder.

3.5 TIPS FOR WOMEN WITH ADHD

When women learn they have dyslexia, they often feel relieved (ADHD). They may have hated themselves for their failures for years, and their consciousness has suffered as a result. Emotional, mental, and bodily fatigue may have resulted from their constant concern over every aspect of their life.

They have an answer now that they have been diagnosed with ADHD, and they recognize that their illnesses are not their fault. Feelings of inadequacy may go away once individuals understand they have ADHD, putting them in a good situation to effectively manage their symptoms.

Symptoms presentation

Women are more likely than males to internalize their symptoms. Girls' symptoms are more focused on inattentiveness and disarray. Families and peers are less likely to be attracted to these symptoms for diagnosis since they are frequently overlooked.

Diagnosing ADHD in Women

The majority of people believe that ADHD is a disease that affects hyperactive schoolboys. Women are frequently not diagnosed until maturity since the way ADHD presents in females does not match this stereotype. Make this your top priority if you suspect you have ADHD but haven't been formally diagnosed. The fact that you've been diagnosed may make you feel better about yourself.

After being diagnosed with ADHD, women seemed able to accept themselves for previous errors and feel more in command of their present circumstances, according to one research. It was great to know they weren't insane, so there was a term for what they had been going through.

Coping strategies

Women may be able to conceal the negative consequences of their ADHD symptoms if they acquire stronger coping mechanisms than their male counterparts. Many people, for example, overcompensate by creating lists to keep themselves organized. While this method is effective, it makes it extremely simple for physicians to overlook the diagnosis.

Women's problems with ADHD may increase as they get older. When the framework of education is no longer tenable, and the actual academic standard is greater, for example, ADHD symptoms may start to create more difficulties.

Comorbid psychiatric disorders

Because females' ADHD symptoms are less disruptive, mood disorders are often identified before they are examined for ADHD. ADHD seldom travels alone. Therefore, you may be suffering from one or more additional illnesses in contrast to your ADHD. Make an effort not to be frightened. Knowing what additional illnesses you may have, if any, enables you to address them individually, allowing you to live the healthiest life. Signs of one disease may sometimes be confused with symptoms of ADHD and vice versa. The majority of people with ADHD would have had at least one comorbid mental illness, which may include:

- Substance abuse disorders
- Anxiety disorders, bipolar disorder, and depression are all examples of anxiety disorders.
- Personality disorders

This is why it's critical to tell your doctor about all of your symptoms and concerns. Being open about your feelings does not imply that you are whining. Your surgeon wants to understand how you're feeling and what you're going through so that they can then provide you with the best treatment possible.

Hyperactivity in Women

Women may be classified with hyperactivity-impulsivity ADHD, but it is less common than inattentive ADHD in women. Hyperactivity comes with its own set of difficulties. You may discover that you have more vitality than your classmates and that you are always chatting. You may recall being rejected, criticized, and ostracized by your classmates because you seemed to be different. This is something that can be carried on into maturity.

3.6 LIVING WITH ADHD

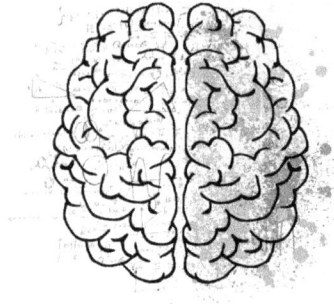

There are a variety of things you may do to help to cope with ADHD symptoms easier.

4

MANAGE YOUR ADHD

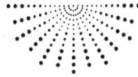

ccepting your ADHD diagnosis, whether you've been diagnosed recently or for years, is a difficult job. You now have a reason why you do things the way you do, and even with the diagnoses, you still have many questions. How so many times have you heard someone remark, "If he wanted to, he could accomplish anything." There'd be no need for ADHD medicines, counseling, or other treatment options if this were the case. The world is a fantastic place to live. The truth is that it isn't that easy. It's essential to "want" to control your ADHD, but studies and experience show that even great desire isn't always enough.

Did you feel unwanted all of the time? Faulty? Apologies? Many people with ADHD suffer from shame as a result of a childhood of self-blame. Learn where it arises from, why it isn't good for you, and how to enhance your social well-being. It may seem like a never-ending flood of apologies when you have ADHD. We're sorry we're late, sorry we misplaced our keys, and sorry that we can't keep the home clean no matter what the situation. These repeated regrets and identity may have built up to a crushing feeling of guilt if you have ADHD, particularly if you were treated late in life. You might have had difficulty managing your guilt if you won't even glance in your bag because you're tormented by how unorganized it is.

It may be difficult to live with ADHD at times. Many people, on the other hand, are able to successfully control their ADHD symptoms and have productive, fulfilling lives. Based on the intensity of your problems, you may not require immediate medical Attention. To gain a grip on your symptoms, you may make a variety of personal changes first.

Despite mounting irrefutable evidence, many individuals continue to deny whether ADHD is a legitimate medical disease. They use it as a justification to be sloppy or lazy. The fact that ADHD seems to come and go depending on the circumstances further adds to the skepticism of the skeptics. They say things like, "Why can't you get it together?" or "Why can't you pull it together?" Why can't you sit down and complete your schoolwork when you're OK with specific friends?"

Another reason is the general disapproval or use of psychotropic medications. The number of individuals using ADHD medication has increased dramatically in recent years. Some question whether the increase is warranted. Finally, the idea that ADHD may have a negative impact on academic achievement exacerbates the stigma. "If your grades are bad, you're not worth anything," our culture appears to believe. This is particularly true if the underlying reason for low performance is unknown, as it is in the case of ADHD.

4.1 MANAGE YOUR ADHD

How so many times have you heard someone remark, "If he wanted to, he could accomplish anything." There'd be no need for ADHD medicines, counseling, or other treatment options if this were the case. The world is a fantastic place to live. The truth is that it isn't that easy. It's essential to "want" to control your ADHD, but studies and experience show that even great desire isn't always enough. To control ADHD, you'll need bravery and a strong desire:

- Diagnosis
- Structure
- Energy
- Education
- Individual Responsibility

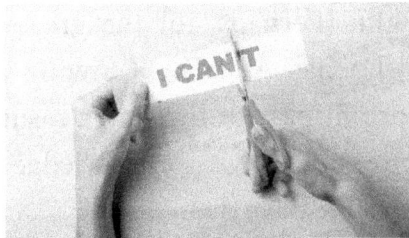

Diagnosis

The initial step toward management is the most significant. Professional diagnosis is an important component of therapy for someone with ADHD. Other diseases require an

accurate diagnosis to get appropriate therapy. Who is quali-
fied to diagnose ADHD? Doctors, psychologists, psychiatrists, and other specialists are educated to identify and
diagnose symptoms.

The sense of relief that follows from just giving the actual
chaos in your life a name is amazing. When people read the
symptoms of ADHD, it's perhaps the only ailment that
makes them smile. Those that do not smile just shake their
heads. "It felt as If I was read about myself" is a common
reaction.

I'm not a lunatic!" you want to scream, "I'm not crazy!" as
you race down the street. Of course, such a display is highly
improper in and of itself, and it may very well convince
people around your that you are completely insane,
prompting them to wrap you in a white shirt and cart you
away for much rest. But, at least, you'll be swept away by the
sense of relief that stems from the fact that the disease that
has brought you so much stress and sorrow has a name.

Energy

Above everything, don't surrender. Battle the good fight
with all you might. (Perhaps not the greatest term to use
with someone who has ADHD.) Knowing about taking a
break is an important part of fighting a losing battle. There
are going to be terrible days. Acknowledge them for how
much they are: terrible days that come now and again. It isn't
the final destination as we know it. Take a step back, gather
your thoughts, and try again.

There are a lot of misunderstandings about ADHD, just
as there are a lot of misconceptions about a lot of other
health problems. These misconceptions are harming the

people in the community about the situation. They may cause issues, including delays in diagnosis and a sense of misunderstanding among patients. According to the Joint Committee of Mental Condition (NAMI), about 9% of children and 4% of adults have ADHD. There's a good chance you know someone who suffers from it.

Structure

For individuals with ADHD, a lack of organization is a significant issue. There appears to be no integrated platform of organizing for most individuals with ADHD. External organizational structures must be created to compensate for the absence of internal structure.

Structure entails more than just remembering where you placed your shoes. Children and adults with ADHD benefit greatly from a structured environment, according to research. So, whether you hire a coach or attempt to do it on your own, finding a method to restore balance to your chaotic world is critical.

Education

Most individuals do extensive studies on ADHD after being diagnosed. People who haven't been able to concentrate on anything before will become highly on reading about ADHD. This is great, but the information must be accurate. There is a great deal of misinformation that is out regarding ADHD.

Individual Responsibility

- Stop blaming others and take a long, hard look in the mirror.
- Accept responsibility for your actions.

- The constant whining of Attitude Deficiency Disorder is much more debilitating than Asperger's Syndrome. Yes, you do have a problem. We'll take care of it.

Accept part of the blame. Make every effort to complete the tasks at hand. When you make a mistake, own up to it, deal with this now, and move on. Teaching a kid that having ADHD absolves them of any repercussions for their behavior simply serves to limit the child's potential.

Treatment for ADHD may be beneficial, but the medication itself will not ensure that you pay your mortgage on time. Finding a method to fulfill your responsibilities and commitments is part of being responsible.

4.2 ACCEPTING YOUR ADHD

Accepting Your Diagnosis

Accepting your ADHD diagnosis, whether you've been diagnosed recently or for years, is a difficult job. You now have a reason why you do things the way you do, and even with the diagnoses, you still have many questions.

- Accept that your neurochemistry is how it is; don't think of it as anything wrong, terrible, or broken with you.
- Recognize that ADHD isn't the most important aspect of your personality. It's simply something about you, and it's not the only thing that comes to mind when somebody thinks of you.

- Recognize that our life continues to have highs and lows, as it has in the past.
- Accepting your ADHD will not make your stress go. ADHD will continue to obstruct your life, but how you speak to yourself about it will vary.

It's critical to comprehend your ADHD before you can completely embrace it.

Understanding your ADHD

If you want to acquire control over your ADHD, you must first understand the condition as much. Consequently, study books, online sites, journals; watch yourself and others in support groups and discuss with experts; your psychiatrists (be nice with them as they are very sensitive!) and coaches; and find out how ADHD affects you. All those with ADHD have various difficulties and have distinct strengths, so learn all about your ADHD.

Understanding entails repairing low self- after decades of criticism, getting fresh insights about what may eventually work for you, and, most crucially, knowledge entails new hope.

You are different

Adults with ADHD get unique neurology that has a wide-ranging and profound impact on their lives. Certain medications may assist. However, there is no cure. Hopefully, as you learn to appreciate both the good and bad aspects of ADHD, you will no longer want a cure. It is entirely possible to have a full, successful, and happy life effectively treating ADHD issues. We suggest that you learn to recognize, acknowledge, and accept your ADHD.

Accepting your ADHD

There seem to be two reasonable options for dealing with our ADHD difficulties and issues, in my opinion. Accepting that we already have a problem and devising an Aids approach or strategic plan to resolve or manage it;

- Accepting that we struggle with that and deciding to live with it and quit fretting ourselves over it;
- Accepting that we find it difficult with something and deciding to live with it and quit worrying ourselves over it; Accepting that we struggle with that and deciding to live with it and quit fretting ourselves over it

Focus on how to keep things interesting, how to build and exploit current habits, how to prevent overload, how to reward oneself, how to discover simpler methods to begin activities and engage yourself, and how to establish the habits and routines to keep doing them.

Embracing your ADHD

Medicine is in the business of identifying and defining disease and treating symptoms with medicines and treatment. With the increasing love of order, regularity, and procedure, ADHD characteristics may make life in today's society challenging. Depression, anxiety, and addictions are all "co-morbidities" of ADHD. Workplace issues, as well as issues with friends and family, may arise. It's wonderful that physicians are engaged in providing medical assistance to individuals with ADHD, but it doesn't make them experts in living a joyful ADHD life.

Shame may result in depressive disorders, debilitating anxiety and, in some instances, self-medication with drink or drugs — all of which will make it more difficult to address issues and break free from the vicious circle. As a result of your shame, you may become defensive, which may come off as anger. If you blow out at those closest to them, you risk alienating them at a time when you need them the most.

Break the Moral Diagnosis

You cannot see shame via this system of ethics to completely overcome it. Instead, consider your Attention from a neurobiological standpoint. Don't think about ADHD as a personal flaw since actual research backs it up, such as MRIs and genetic studies. Recognize that although the disease does exist, it is not a flaw; it is just an issue of brain chemicals. It's your task to meet, and it's up to you to figure out how to do so.

Confronting the Skeptics

Nevertheless, some people still consider ADHD a moral flaw and people with ADHD to be slackers. You've probably absorbed the critical murmurs if you've heard them throughout your life. "My issue seems to be that I lack patience," you think as you peer inside your cluttered purse. You lash out for yourself when you're late for yet another meeting: "I'm a shambles." I have a bad habit of being lazy. "There's no way I'm going to get ahead."

Adopt a Strength-Based Approach

Instead of focusing on the bad aspects of your ADHD, embrace the good aspects. Please take a moment to consider your skills and qualities whenever guilt rears its ugly head. Creativity, initiative, perseverance, inventiveness, and other

traits are associated with ADHD. Even when it seems difficult, learn to identify these characteristics in yourself. You'll
be better able to fight yourself against emotions of shame if
you strive to bring them out and develop them.

You are not Alone

Don't allow your location to get in the way of your
success! And do not be hesitant to seek assistance from a
professional, a friend, or even your spouse. Having individuals on your staff that "get them" and are on the lookout for
you may be very beneficial. Many therapists provide Skype
or phone appointments, and online service groups may help
you feel connected no matter where you are.

Expect Respect

Shame-stricken people are prone to allowing others to
walk everywhere around them. You may be scared to argue
with your employer because you're frightened of saying
something foolish. However, this is a personality prophecy:
if you don't expect respect, you won't get it. Instead of being
hindered through shame, you may establish healthy bound-
aries for how others treat you when you learn to appreciate
your talents.

Anti-shame systems

Face your sorrow straight on, addressing the problems
that are causing it. In contrast, if you're embarrassed because
you often misplace your vehicle keys, devise a method to stay
on top of them. Try placing a little basket on a table near the
front entrance and training yourself to throw your vehicle
keys in it every time you come in. As your history improves,
your guilt will give way to pride and a greater sense of self-
worth.

Don't give up

People living with ADHD are very tenacious. It's the thing that makes them unique that they try harder, even when it's difficult. You may strive to put your shame back after you've identified your good qualities, built your supportive relationship, and discovered where you flourish.

5

ADHD, MEDIATION AND HOLISTIC EATING HABITS

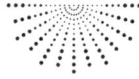

M edications and counseling may help you manage the symptoms of ADHD. They aren't, however, your sole choices. Mindfulness meditation, in which you actively notice your moment-to-moment emotions and emotions, may now be a useful method to quiet your mind and increase your concentration, according to new research. This technique is used by and over a third of people with ADHD, and approximately 40% of them rate it highly.

Mindfulness meditation, unlike other therapies, does not need medication or a visit to a doctor's office. It may be done while sitting, walking, or even doing certain kinds of yoga. Do you have an overabundance of thoughts going through your head? Consider a sky that is blue with white fluffy clouds. The clouds symbolize your ideas, while the sky symbolizes your consciousness. To refocus your attention, concentrate on the "space" between the clouds. If you have difficulty keeping still, walking meditation may be just as effective as seated meditation. Bring your focus back to the feelings on the bottoms of your feet when your mind wanders.

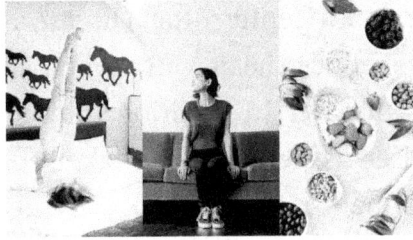

Developing excellent everyday life management skills is an important part of gaining control of ADHD. These abilities will assist you in taking control of your everyday life, making effective usage of your time, learning how to break and achieve bigger life objectives, and developing daily routines that will improve well-being and decrease ADHD symptoms.

We should start developing these abilities while we are teenagers so that our shift to an independent life is easier. These abilities include knowing how to organize your time, prioritize and recall your daily chores, and also developing healthy daily routines such as getting enough sleep, exercising regularly, and eating properly. As an ADHD sufferer, your aim is to do all you can to enhance your brain's functioning, and sleep, diet, and exercise may help you achieve that goal by balancing your brain chemistry and improving your mood and concentration.

A healthy, well-balanced diet is essential for a happy & healthy existence. A balanced diet may help alleviate some of the symptoms of ADHD when used in conjunction with other treatments. Taking an objective look at your eating habits and determining what works well for you and your kid, on the other hand, maybe a difficult task. Eating correctly, as per the Centers for Disease and Prevention (CDC), may help reduce the risk of several chronic illnesses, especially heart disease. In addition, physical activity and exercise are advised as elements of a balanced lifestyle.

Dietary treatments for ADHD include removing or reducing one or more items from a person's meal (for example, candy, sugar and food with red dye). The idea is that dietary sensitivities may induce or exacerbate ADHD symptoms. However, careful study has shown that this method is not effective as a therapy.

Nutritional supplements and high dosages of vitamins may complement a diet that some people feel is lacking. Some individuals believe that taking dietary supplements may help with ADHD symptoms. This theory has yet to be proven by scientists.

5.1 MEDITATION AND YOGA FOR ADHD

Medications and counseling may help you manage the symptoms of ADHD. They aren't, however, your sole choices. Mindfulness meditation, in which you actively notice your moment-to-moment emotions and emotions, may now be a useful method to quiet your mind and increase your concentration, according to new research. This technique is used by and over a third of people with ADHD, and approximately 40% of them rate it highly.

Mindfulness meditation, unlike other therapies, does not need medication or a visit to a doctor's office. It may be done while sitting, walking, or even doing certain kinds of yoga.

How does It work?

When a specific muscle is weak, you can do exercises to make it stronger. The same may be said about your mind. Meditation that focuses on mindfulness improves your capacity to manage your attention. It shows you how to look at yourself in the mirror and concentrate on something. It also shows you how to pull your wandering mind back to the present. It may also assist you in being more aware of your emotions, rendering you less likely to act rashly. Meditation is thought to help with ADHD therapy by expanding the prefrontal cortex, a brain area involved in attention, planning, and impulse control. It also boosts dopamine levels in the brain, which are low in ADHD patients' brains.

According to research, mindfulness meditation may assist those with ADHD symptoms. People having ADHD who attended a 2-1/2-hour mindfulness meditation class once a week for 8 weeks, then performed a regular home meditation practice that progressively grew from 5 to 15 minutes, were better able to remain focused on activities, according to a major UCLA research. They were also fewer worried and sad. Since then, several investigations have shown similar findings.

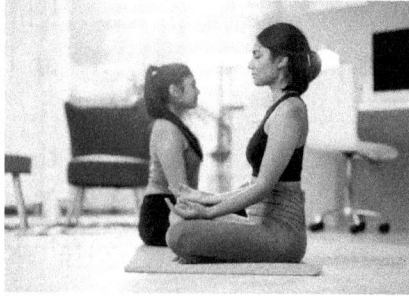

Although much of the study has been conducted with children, yoga has been proven to help alleviate ADHD symptoms. It increases dopamine levels and improves the prefrontal brain, much like mindfulness meditation. According to one research, children who performed yoga movements for 20 minutes two times a week for eight weeks improved on attention and concentration assessments.

Other Benefits

This kind of relaxation method may benefit individuals with ADHD in addition to alleviating their symptoms:

- Increase self-esteem
- Reduce fat
- Reduce anxiety

People with ADHD are often harsh on themselves since they have difficulty getting things completed on time and maybe forgetful. However, you may employ meditation to silence the critical voice in your mind.

When people practice mindfulness meditation on a regular basis, their stress hormone levels are shown to be lower in situations or circumstances that induce anxiety, such as when they feel powerless and out of control. Mindfulness meditation has also been linked to weight loss, perhaps because it causes you to look more critically about anything you do, such as what you consume.

Tips for Meditating with ADHD

Do you have an overabundance of thoughts going through your head? Consider a sky that is blue with white fluffy clouds. The clouds symbolize your ideas, while the sky symbolizes your consciousness. To refocus your attention, concentrate on the "space" between the clouds. If you have difficulty keeping still, walking meditation may be just as effective as seated meditation. Bring your focus back to the feelings on the bottoms of your feet when your mind wanders.

• Having someone to practice meditation and yoga with may help you stay with it, much as having a friend to keep your companionship during exercises can help you continue with it.

• Make some signals to assist you in making it a habit. Make a note of it in your calendar, or set a reminder on your phone at a particular time.

• Sitting motionless may seem to be all that meditation entails. Meditation, on the other hand, is a proactive practice that teaches the brain to concentrate and be present.

When you or your kid suffers from ADHD (attention deficit hyperactivity disorder), meditation may appear difficult. However, studies show that individuals with ADHD may effectively meditate and that mindfulness may help with a few of the behaviors linked with ADHD. Here are eight suggestions to assist you or your kid practice to relax and control ADHD-related behaviors.

6

ADHD TREATMENT OPTIONS

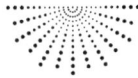

The individual's specific requirements are emphasized when it relates to therapy for any psychiatric condition. Discuss your worries, questions, and preferences with the members of your therapy team to decide which method is best for you, and inquire about the many choices available.

Adults with ADHD often get treatment in the form of medication, counseling, skill development, and appropriate accommodations.

Loved ones and important others may benefit from marriage counseling or family therapy to help them deal with the stress of life with somebody who has ADHD. It may also educate kids on how to assist and how to communicate more effectively with another person. ADHD is treated with stimulant and non-stimulant medicines. Stimulants are recommended as the first line of therapy. They aid in the regulation of norepinephrine and dopamine, different chemical messengers in the brain.

People often seek remedies for ADHD (attention deficit hyperactivity disorder) that people think will work in conjunction with and instead of the therapies prescribed by their doctor. Physicians and many others cure ADHD utilizing techniques that have been thoroughly researched, tested, and shown to be successful. Medication and behavioral therapy are two of these approaches. There are, however, a slew of alternative ADHD therapies that individuals hear about from colleagues or read about on the internet.

Is it any surprise that people having attention deficit hyperactivity disorder (ADHD and ADD) have dangerously low self-esteem and constant negative thoughts after a lifetime of errors, accidents, and missed deadlines? Cognitive-behavioral therapy is goal-oriented, short-term psychotherapy that seeks to alter negative thought habits and improve how a person thinks regarding herself, her skills, as well as her prospects. Call it ADHD brain therapy.

CBT is founded on cognitive reorganization or the understanding that cognitions contribute to emotional problems. It was first developed as a therapy for mood disorders. Automatic ideas are interpretations of events that occur without prompting. Unfounded preconceptions regarding yourself (and others), a circumstance, or the future, for example, may alter these perceptions. Such negative mental dialogues make it difficult for a person to strive for a specific goal, establish new productive habits, or take calculated risks.

CBT attempts to alter illogical thinking processes that make it difficult for people to remain on target or complete tasks. CBT challenges the reality of a person with ADHD who believes, "This needs to be flawless, or it's no good," or "I never accomplish anything properly." Treatment for anxiety and other emotional disorders involves changing erroneous beliefs and the consequent changes in behavior patterns.

6.1 THERAPY FOR ADHD

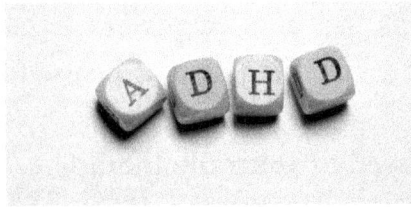

Adult ADHD therapy may be helpful. It usually includes psychiatric therapy as well as information on the illness. Therapy can help you:

- learn ways of managing impulsive behavior
- improve one's time management and organizational skills
- develop strategies to manage your temper
- cope with school or work difficulties
- create connections with your family, coworkers, and friends
- boost your self-esteem
- learn better issue solving skills

Adults with ADHD may benefit from a variety of therapies, including:

- cognitive-behavioral therapy (CBT)
- marriage counseling or family therapy

Cognitive-behavioral therapy (CBT)

CBT (cognitive behavioral therapy) teaches you how to control your behavior and transform negative ideas into good ones. It may also assist you in dealing with issues in your relationships, in school, or at work.

Individual or group therapy may be used for this kind of treatment.

Marital counseling or family therapy

Loved ones and important others may benefit from marriage counseling or family therapy to help them deal with the stress of life with somebody who has ADHD. It may also educate kids on how to assist and how to communicate more effectively with another person.

Medications for ADHD

The most common stimulants given to people with ADHD are:

- dextroamphetamine (Dexedrine)
- amphetamine salts (Adderall XR, Maydays)
- Lisdexamfetamine (Vyvanse)

These drugs work by increasing and regulating the amounts of neurotransmitters in the brain, which assist in managing ADHD symptoms.

Atomoxetine (Strattera) and some antidepressants, such as bupropion, are two more medicines that may be used to treat ADHD (Wellbutrin). Antidepressants and atomoxetine act more slowly than stimulants. Thus, symptoms may take many weeks to improve.

- The appropriate medicine and dosage are frequently different from one individual to the next. Finding what works best for you may take a little time at first.
- To ensure that you are completely informed, speak to a doctor about the advantages and dangers of each drug.
- If you have any adverse effects while taking your medicine, you should contact your doctor.
- ADHD may create difficulties in personal relations and impair school performance or job if it is not identified and addressed.

It's not easy to have ADHD as an adult. You may, however, significantly decrease your symptoms and enhance your life quality with the proper therapy and lifestyle changes.

6.2 ADULT ADHD MEDICATIONS

ADHD is treated with stimulant and non-stimulant medicines. Stimulants are recommended as the first line of therapy. They aid in the regulation of norepinephrine and dopamine, different chemical messengers in the brain.

7

MANAGING RELATIONSHIPS AND WORK WITH ADHD

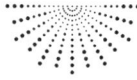

M any people heard of attention deficit hyperactivity disorder (ADHD), which is some-times known as attention deficit (ADD), albeit this is an obsolete name. Many individuals may be familiar with the word, but they are unsure of what it includes or what it means. Attention deficit hyperactivity disorder (ADHD) is an acronym for attention deficit hyperactivity disorder. This implies that your spouse may exhibit focus problems as well as hyperactive habits. This neurodevelop-mental condition is persistent, which means it lasts for the rest of a human's body. Most of us are familiar with the symptoms of attention deficit disorder (ADHD) in children: fidgety, hyperactive, difficulty getting organized, and lack of concentration. According to the Depression Association of America, around 60% of children with ADHD continue to experience symptoms throughout adulthood. That's approximately 8 million people or 1.3 million of the adult population.

Adults with ADHD have a somewhat distinct appearance. It may manifest as agitation, disorganization, and difficulty concentrating. ADHD may also have some distinct advantages. Adult ADHD professionals may find that choosing a job that capitalizes on their abilities rather than relying primarily on weak spots is the key to a personal career. That, as well as effective ADHD therapy.

Listening carefully, being able to empathize with the person you're speaking to, and then acting in a helpful, non-defensive manner are all essential components of good communication. It also entails expressing your own ideas and emotions in a non-judgmental or accusatory manner so that your other partner can really hear and comprehend what you're saying rather than getting enraged or defensive. Stay calm, listen, empathize, react, and problem-solve; this may seem easy and uncomplicated. When emotions take control, however, excellent communication skills are frequently forgotten as partners participate in denials, accusations, refusals to resume talking, interruptions, and a variety of other behavior that obstruct healthy communication.

Adults with ADHD have even more communication difficulties since ADHD impulsivity may create disruptions even when emotions are low, and ADHD distractibility can cause your mind to wander just as your spouse is telling you something extremely important to him or her. As they're so focused on the ideas they are attempting to convey, somebody with ADHD may miss nonverbal signals that their companion is getting upset. Many people with ADHD have poor emotional self-control, making them highly and the over to even moderately unpleasant remarks.

Those with ADHD may seem indifferent to their partner's demands while they are engrossed in the difficulties of their own everyday lives. It's awful to be late for work, a doctor's appointment, a meeting, a friend's birthday party, bringing the child to college, and much worse, picking them up from school. What can you do to break the cycle? How can you better manage your time? Experts say that successful planning requires two abilities that individuals with ADHD typically lack naturally but may learn: planning and timing.

7.1 THE EFFECTS OF ADULT ADHD ON RELATIONSHIPS

Anyone may find it difficult to form and sustain a solid connection. Having ADHD, on the other hand, may provide a variety of difficulties. Partners may see them as:

- preoccupied partners or parents
- poor listeners
- forgetful due to this neurodevelopmental condition.

Unfortunately, these most loving relationships may fail because of such problems. Understanding how adult ADHD affects relationships may help you avoid having a bad relationship. In reality, there are methods to guarantee that your partnership is totally joyful.

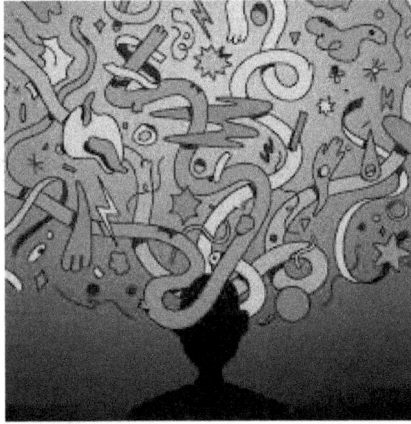

Understanding ADHD

Many people heard of attention deficit hyperactivity disorder (ADHD), which is sometimes known as attention deficit (ADD), albeit this is an obsolete name. Many individuals may be familiar with the word, but they are unsure of what it includes or what it means. Attention deficit hyperactivity disorder (ADHD) is an acronym for attention deficit hyperactivity disorder. This implies that your spouse may exhibit focus problems as well as hyperactive habits. This neurodevelopmental condition is persistent, which means it lasts for the rest of a human's body.

The majority of individuals struggle with the following:

- a lack of drive
- time management
- a lack of focus
- problems with organization

- self-control

The spouse with ADHD may have furious or inappropriate outbursts in their relationships. Unpleasant situations may sometimes erupt, causing stress to spouses and children. Although these outbursts of rage may pass quickly, harsh comments said on the spur of the moment may create stress in the household.

ADHD and Relationship Difficulties

Despite the fact that each spouse carries their own luggage into a marriage, a person with ADHD is often burdened with the following points:

- a lack of self-assurance
- a poor self-image
- humiliation from previous "failures."

Their propensity to lavish their lover with passion and attention, a characteristic of ADHD hyperfocus, may disguise these problems at first.

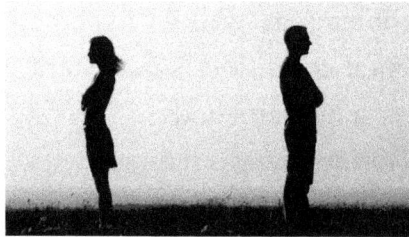

However, the hyper focus's focus eventually changes. When this happens, an individual with ADHD may appear to pay little attention to their spouse. This may cause the neglected spouse to question whether they are truly loved. A relationship may be strained as a result of this dynamic. The ADHD spouse may continuously doubt their partner's love or devotion, which may be misinterpreted as a loss of integrity. This may cause the marriage to become even more estranged.

ADHD and Marriage

ADHD may put even greater pressure on a relationship. As the year's pass, the partner who is not afflicted by ADHD discovers that they are responsible for the majority of:

- domestic responsibilities
- financial accountability
- parenting
- household management
- dealing with family issues

Because of this division of responsibilities, the ADHD partner may seem to be a kid rather than a mate. The sexual dynamic weakens if the marriage becomes a parent-child connection. The non-ADHD partner may see their partner's actions as a symbol of affection lost. Divorce is a possibility in this scenario.

Empathy is crucial if your partner suffers from ADHD. Take some deep breaths and recall why you fell in love when things become difficult. Small reminders like this may help you get through even the most stressful days. If you think like you can't handle it any longer, marital therapy may be a good option.

Why Breakups Happen

The separation may come as a total surprise to the ADHD spouse, who was too preoccupied to see that the partnership was deteriorating. The spouse with ADHD may have emotionally and mentally retreated in an attempt to avoid feeling overwhelmed by chores or demanding children, leaving the other spouse feeling deserted and resentful.

This dynamic is exacerbated if the ADHD spouse is untreated and not receiving treatment. Even yet, therapy may not be enough to alleviate rage and bitterness. The longer a relationship's issues are ignored, the more likely it is to end in divorce.

Considering Couples Therapy

If a couple dealing with ADHD wants to save their relationship, they must understand that ADHD, not the individual with the disease, is the issue. Blame one another for ADHD's adverse effects will only deepen the divide between them. The following are some of the possible negative effects:

- a cluttered home
- a reduction in sex life
- financial difficulties

At the very least, the ADHD partner should be treated with medication and therapy. Couples counseling with an ADHD specialist may offer extra support for both spouses and help the couple get back to constructive, honest communication. Couples who manage the condition together may assist each other in repairing their connections and take on constructive roles in their relationship.

Relationships may be harmed by ADHD; however, this is not the case. Mutual acceptance of flaws may go a long way toward building empathy for one another and teaching people to slow down.

Compassion and cooperation are at the top of the list of characteristics that make an ADHD partner relationship succeed. At some moment, you should urge your spouse to get therapy if you believe it will help to alleviate some of the more severe symptoms. Counseling may also help you develop the teamwork skills you both need.

A relationship with someone who has ADHD is never simple, but it isn't destined to fail either. The following therapy may help you maintain a good and healthy relationship:

- medication
- attempts to improve communication
- counseling
- mutual respect for one another
- dedication to a fair distribution of duties

7.2 BEST JOBS FOR PEOPLE WITH ADHD

Most of us are familiar with the symptoms of attention deficit disorder (ADHD) in children: fidgety, hyperactive, difficulty getting organized, and lack of concentration. According to the Depression Association of America, around 60% of children with ADHD continue to experience symptoms throughout adulthood. That's approximately 8 million people or 1.3 million of the adult population.

Adults with ADHD have a somewhat distinct appearance. It may manifest as agitation, disorganization, and difficulty concentrating. ADHD may also have some distinct advantages. Adult ADHD professionals may find that choosing a job that capitalizes on their abilities rather than relying primarily on weak spots is the key to a personal career. That, as well as effective ADHD therapy.

Some people with ADHD may benefit from certain work characteristics:

- Passion-driven
- Self-starter
- Ultra-structured
- High-intensity
- Lightning-fast
- Hands-on creative

Finding a profession that excels in one or more of these characteristics, or a mix of all, maybe the key to a fulfilling career. Take a look at these positions that may be a good match for you.

High-intensity
Jobs

Investigator, policeman, critical care physician, correctional officer, emergency dispatch, sports coach, and fireman are just a few of the jobs available.

Jobs with just an inherent feeling of urgency typically succeed for individuals with ADHD because they are driven by intensity. Careers, where a person's life is at stake, offer the most intense feeling of urgency.

People with ADHD thrive in high-intensity, fast-paced environments, such as an emergency department or an ambulance.

Passion-fueled Jobs

Writer, doctor, registered nurse, veterinarian, caseworker, fitness trainer, spiritual clergy, psychiatrist, high school teacher, writer, doctor, registered nurse

Jobs that require you to be extremely enthusiastic in what you do offer a natural source of drive and concentration. This may be an area in which you have a strong and long-lasting interest. The possibilities are endless.

Ultra-structured Jobs

Military, project leader, data scientist, lawyer, software tester, lawyer, property insurance adjuster, bank teller, and factory assembly line worker are just a few of the jobs available.

Some people with ADHD thrive in employment with a lot of structure. A structured job has a set process, routine, and duties that are well defined. There isn't much room for interpretation, and there are no expectations.

According to Children and People with Attention-Deficit/Hyperactivity Disorder, time management may be one of the most difficult parts of work for adults with ADHD.

Jobs with building and regularity may help you succeed in your career. Employees with ADHD flourish in settings that provide them with clear instructions and directions. It entails a lot of meticulously following checklists and repeatedly performing technical processes.

Hands-on creative
Jobs

Designer, clothing designer, engineer, graphic artist, interior decorator, architect, musician, artist, dancer, entertainment For some individuals with ADHD, hands-on occupations that demand creativity are ideal. These professions often involve creativity and problem-solving, two skills that individuals with ADHD thrive at.

People with ADHD often have little sense of achieving greater levels of creative thinking and achievement, according to research. Those rushing thoughts and ideas may often be transformed into brilliant creative thinking and production.

Lightning pace
Jobs

ER nurse, traumatic doctor/surgeon, EMT, fireman, schoolteacher, dental assistant, and retail clerk are all examples of people who work in the emergency room.

Constant and fast-changing thoughts are one of the characteristics of ADHD. Using such a skill may lead to professional success. Many people with ADHD say that they like continuous change or thrive in situations that require them to evaluate and adjust rapidly.

Independent risk-taker
Jobs

A brokerage firm, pro athlete, businessman, commercial diver, construction supervisor, software designer, racing car driver, and aircraft pilot are all examples of people who work in the financial industry.

Some individuals with ADHD possess two skills: a desire to take chances and the ability to think creatively. These qualities may help you thrive as a self-employed person or in professions that need a lot of freedom. Because occupations demanding independence frequently require mastering skills that individuals with ADHD have trouble with, including planning, organizing, and self-motivation, the work must be in a subject you're enthusiastic about.

7.3 ADHD MANAGEMENT TOOLS

Keeping organized is a difficult task, and people with ADHD may need more assistance than others.

Task planner and calendar

Aside from the apparent benefit of remembering meetings and obligations, utilizing this application on a regular basis allows you to do 2 factors:

- scheduling things over time; this is a difficult job for many individuals with ADHD.
- Overcome "big project overload" by breaking down larger activities into smaller ones

Writing things down may also make you feel more successful since it enables you to visually cross items off your list and see how far you've progressed.

Command center

A logistical headquarters is required in every household. Look for ideas on Pinterest that are appropriate for your situation. Set aside a space, ideally close to the entrance, for a:

- Use a whiteboard to convey essential information.
- Drop-off and pick-up location for keys, papers, handbags, children's backpacks, library books, incoming laundry service, and other essentials

AFTERWORD

ADHD is a neurobiological disease, which means it affects the biology of the central nervous and is characterized by impairments in executive functioning and self-control. Inattention, ADHD, or a mix of the two are the outcomes. To be diagnosed with ADHD, the condition must have begun in childhood and be causing impairment in one or more settings. Let's take a closer look at the consequences of executive dysfunction.

Every single one of us has struggled with the opening sentence of a dissertation or an essential letter at one point or another. The road to getting past the mental stalemate is not always smooth, but many of us eventually managed to summon this same complex planning and organizational skills required to write term papers or manage work projects or to plan a kitchen renovation or separate dark from the light-colored laundry at some point. The three kinds of

ADHD are ADD (often referred to as ADD or attention deficit disorder).

Though the overwhelming majority of instances of ADHD are hereditary, it is possible to develop ADHD as a result of brain damage, sickness, or perinatal exposure to harmful chemicals in rare circumstances. It's essential to remember ADHD isn't caused by bad parenting, too much TV, or a poor diet. We've probably heard the misconceptions about ADHD: "ADHD isn't real." "That child only needs a really good spanking," says the narrator. "Individuals having ADHD are simply lazy."

These misunderstandings and falsehoods regarding ADHD have existed since the disease itself; the detrimental impact on people's lives is quite real and extremely harmful. Find out the reality and equip yourself with evidence to counter the next ignorant remark about "poor parenting." Despite breakthrough research and unambiguous neurobiological results, many individuals continue to hold incorrect ideas about ADHD, and some even propagate outright falsehoods, which only serve to perpetuate confusion, shame and stigma.

Behavioral problems (ADHD) affect two-thirds of children and will continue to affect them as adults. Although adults are calmer, they still struggle with organization and impulsivity. Some ADHD medicines for youngsters may help manage symptoms that persist into adulthood. ADHD's impact on sexuality may be difficult to quantify. This is because each person's sexual symptoms may vary. Sexual dysfunction may be caused by certain sexual symptoms. This may put a lot of strain on a relationship. Understanding how

ADHD impacts sexuality may help a couple of deal with stress in their relationship.

Women with ADHD have a hard time achieving orgasm. Some women claim to be able to have multiple orgasms in a short period, while others claim to be unable to achieve orgasm despite extended stimulation.

Approximately 80% of people with ADHD will be diagnosed with at least one additional mental illness at some point in their lives. Learning difficulties, anxiety, depression, sensory disorder, and conduct disorder are the most frequent ADHD comorbidities.

Even though women and girls are now more often diagnosed with ADHD, women continue to encounter challenges getting an appropriate diagnosis. Only a few psychiatrists have been trained to diagnose women with ADHD. Because 95% of females having ADHD also have a coexisting illness including stress, anxiety, and bipolar disorder, their difficulties are frequently ascribed to their existing disease, whereas ADHD goes undiagnosed. Another obstacle to female ADHD diagnosis is the absence of obvious symptoms of ADHD in childhood. To establish a diagnosis, current diagnostic standards need evidence of ADHD before the age of seven. Because females with ADHD are lesser prone to have been impulsive, disruptive, or rebellious as children, they are less prone to have been diagnosed with ADHD. Updated ADHD recommendations, set to be released in 2014, don't need early childhood symptoms. Many women will have to overcome this hurdle to identification until then.

Do you imagine a hyperactive young kid climbing the walls when you think of someone with ADHD? Quite a few individuals do. However, this isn't the full picture. ADHD may also manifest itself in the form of a 30-year-old lady securely planted on the sofa. Women with ADHD have a particular list of symptoms and difficulties and coping with the typical pleasures of the disease. Understanding them may help you feel less guilty and confused about being an untidy little woman in a society that demands perfection. When women learn they have dyslexia, they often feel relieved (ADHD). They may have hated themselves for their failures for years, and their consciousness has suffered as a result. Emotional, mental, and bodily fatigue may have resulted from their constant concern over every aspect of their life.

They have an answer now that they have been diagnosed with ADHD, and they recognize that their illnesses are not their fault. Feelings of inadequacy may go away once individuals understand they have ADHD, putting them in a good situation to effectively manage their symptoms.

Accepting your ADHD diagnosis, whether you've been diagnosed recently or for years, is a difficult job. You now have a reason why you do things the way you do, and even with the diagnoses, you still have many questions. How so many times have you heard someone remark, "If he wanted to, he could accomplish anything." There'd be no need for ADHD medicines, counseling, or other treatment options if this were the case. The world is a fantastic place to live. The truth is that it isn't that easy. It's essential to "want" to control your ADHD, but studies and experience show that even great desire isn't always enough.

Did you feel unwanted all of the time? Faulty? Apologies? Many people with ADHD suffer from shame as a result of a childhood of self-blame. Learn where it arises from, why it isn't good for you, and how to enhance your social well-being. It may seem like a never-ending flood of apologies when you have ADHD. We're sorry we're late, sorry we misplaced our keys, and sorry that we can't keep the home clean no matter what the situation. These repeated regrets and identity may have built up to a crushing feeling of guilt if you have ADHD, particularly if you were treated late in life. You might have had difficulty managing your guilt if you won't even glance in your bag because you're tormented by how unorganized it is.

It may be difficult to live with ADHD at times. Many people, on the other hand, are able to successfully control their ADHD symptoms and have productive, fulfilling lives. Based on the intensity of your problems, you may not require immediate medical attention. To gain a grip on your symptoms, you may make a variety of personal changes first.

Developing excellent everyday life management skills is an important part of gaining control of ADHD. These abilities will assist you in taking control of your everyday life, making effective usage of your time, learning how to break and achieve bigger life objectives, and developing daily routines that will improve well-being and decrease ADHD symptoms.

We should start developing these abilities while we are teenagers so that our shift to an independent life is easier. These abilities include knowing how to organize your time, prioritize and recall your daily chores, and also developing healthy daily routines such as getting enough sleep, exercising regularly, and eating properly. As an ADHD sufferer, your aim is to do all you can to enhance your brain's functioning, and sleep, diet, and exercise may help you achieve that goal by balancing your brain chemistry and improving your mood and concentration.

A healthy, well-balanced diet is essential for a happy & healthy existence. A balanced diet may help alleviate some of the symptoms of ADHD when used in conjunction with other treatments. Taking an objective look at your eating habits and determining what works well for you and your kid, on the other hand, maybe a difficult task. Eating correctly, as per the Centers for Disease and Prevention (CDC), may help reduce the risk of several chronic illnesses, especially heart disease. In addition, physical activity and exercise are advised as elements of a balanced lifestyle.

Dietary treatments for ADHD include removing or reducing one or more items from a person's meal (for example, candy, sugar and food with red dye). The idea is that dietary sensitivities may induce or exacerbate ADHD symptoms. However, careful study has shown that this method is not effective as a therapy. In the end, what matters is that ADHD is completely manageable, and we have to put the work in.

CPSIA information can be obtained
at www.ICGtesting.com
Printed in the USA
BVHW040852061221
623325BV00017B/811

9 781739 879822